# KEVIN

## S.M. FLANAGAN

This edition first published in paperback by
Michael Terence Publishing in 2023
www.mtp.agency

Copyright © 2023 S.M. Flanagan

S.M. Flanagan has asserted the right to be identified as
the author of this work in accordance with the
Copyright, Designs and Patents Act 1988

ISBN 9781800945067

No part of this publication may be reproduced, stored
in a retrieval system, or transmitted, in any form or
by any means, electronic, mechanical, photocopying,
recording or otherwise, without the prior
permission of the publisher

Cover image
Copyright © Prapataowsakorn
www.123rf.com

Cover design
Copyright © 2023 Michael Terence Publishing

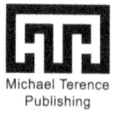

Michael Terence
Publishing

# CONTENTS

THE PSYCHIATRIC PATIENT'S ADMITTANCE ............ 1

PROLOGUE ............ 3

1: KEVIN'S DETENTION ............ 7

2: DAYDREAMER ............ 9

3: KEVIN'S FOOTBALL DISAPPOINTMENTS ............ 14

4: KEVIN SUFFERS WITH MISERY ............ 16

5: PATTY FORCES HER SON TO TIDY UP BEDROOM ... 18

6: KEVIN'S OBSESSIONAL FAVOURITES ............ 20

7: MUSIC LAST PERIOD ............ 21

8: LONELINESS ............ 23

9: LOSING HER COOL, GRANDMOTHER REPRIMANDED KEVIN ............ 25

10: KEVIN'S DESIRE ............ 27

11: KEVIN'S NERVOUS BREAKDOWNS TO HIS FINAL CONVERSION ............ 28

# THE PSYCHIATRIC PATIENT'S ADMITTANCE

Kevin a psychiatric inpatient, a schizophrenic was bewildered, confused and deranged. Kevin felt vulnerable and exposed.

Where was he? What was he doing here? Suffering from claustrophobia. The patient was confined to the sitting area in a ward. The other patients remained in confinement under observation by members of staff on duty.

Kevin remained claustrophobic from remaining confined. Frantically, he read a Bible. The patient felt fearful and frightened. His ignorance of witchcraft (The Black Arts) and the state of his vulnerability and his psychiatric condition were the main factors, in the diagnosis of his schizophrenia.

Kevin stayed sane. He overcame his possession condition by reading the Bible. The patient was feeling weak and fragile. The patient stayed confined in a Psychiatric Ward under observational supervision.

When feeling slightly better, Kevin got dressed and went to the Chapel. There he approached a Priest. Feeling afraid, Kevin asked the Priest a question,

"How do you deal with witchcraft?" asked Kevin.

The Chaplain answered matter-of-factly,

"Do take Holy Communion."

Kevin listened to the experienced Priest. Did this Priest practise exorcism? An Exorcist?

Day after day, Kevin read his Bible and prayed for survival. Kevin survived. Kevin gained deliverance from possession!

Despite Kevin still being under section, the patient had been subjected to Blood Tests administered to him.

On certain times for visiting hours at the Hospital, his Mother and Sister visited Kevin in Hospital. The visitors saw patients whom they visited at Hospital.

Subsequently, Kevin developed self-control, discipline and mortification from reading the scriptures from the Holy Bible every day. From praying and worshipping. A worshipful Kevin did worship.

Consequently, Kevin became less and less afraid as the final week progressed. Finally, the patient was discharged from Hospital. This patient was referred to as an outpatient.

At home, the patient recovered and recuperated. Though Kevin was susceptible to a relapse. Unfortunately, another nervous breakdown. The relapser deteriorated. The Psychiatric Patient was sectioned at Hospital again.

# PROLOGUE

Kevin was once an Irish schoolboy growing up. The schoolboy was rough, tough and decadent. At secondary school, the schoolboy fancied a Female pupil. But this schoolgirl undesired him. Finding him undesirable!

Again, Kevin felt heartrendingly disappointed.

Kevin had no hope of passing his exams. AN EXAMINATION CERTIFICATE FAILURE.

The next year, Kevin enrolled in the Sixth Form. (There he spent his time in a Common Room.)

The Sixth Former ended up failing his Examinations again.

In the Autumn, Kevin enrolled for college. Kevin failed his Examinations again!

Kevin was unemployed. Kevin had no future prospects. His prospects of Further Education and any employment remained negative and pessimistic. From failure, humiliation, frustration and embarrassment Kevin suffered with his miseries!

Kevin become depressed, miserable, violent and dreadfully unhappy.

To pass his time away, Kevin watched video nasties. Actually, watching them made him become sinful, corrupt, depraved and prurient. His way of life seemed to be decadent in those days.

One summer afternoon, an attractive witch came over to his Mother's house. They both talked for a short time. The witch invited Kevin to her house. There Kevin met Erica's Husband and their two sons. Many minutes later, Kevin met Erica's friend's teenage daughter. A playful Teenager with a childish girlishness.

Suddenly, Kevin became possessed! In his state of mind, he was assailed with possession. An insanity! In his mind, Kevin went insane. In his state, he went berserk.

Erica witnessing and seeing Kevin in this state had decided to take Kevin home. Erica's nonchalant girlfriend a stunning Brunette came with her. The passenger accompanying Kevin going insane.

From that day on, Kevin never saw either of them ever again!

At home, Kevin went insane. Reading his pocket Bible frantically. On the verge of a nervous breakdown. Kevin had been bedridden. He tried to jump out of the window to try and get out on a roof to escape. His evil, violent older brother pulled him back in. His brother assaulted him.

Becoming insane, Kevin lost awareness of everything. He was oblivious to everything else.

With his Mother, a weird, coloured man took Kevin in his van.

In his bad state, he was admitted to Hospital in a ward. Subsequently, the admitted patient was sectioned, drugged up and had to have a number of blood tests done against his will.

Day after day, Kevin was pacified by reading his pocket Bible.

During their shifts, a few Professional Nurses attended to the patient. The Uniformed Nurses and also a fashionable, Professional Nurse nursed the patient back to good health, by attending to the patient.

During that time the patient recuperated and convalesced during his stay at Hospital in a Psychiatric Ward. Finally, the patient was discharged from Hospital. This patient was referred to Outpatients.

At home, Kevin recovered. Trying to get back to normality. To pass time away, Kevin would write to occupy himself. He developed a skill for writing. Kevin being unaware was assailed by forces of darkness. Perhaps witchcraft?

Sometime the next year, Kevin's friend suddenly died. His cause of death was cancer. Kevin was shocked by his death. Kevin remained in a state of shock.

Kevin felt so sad, and mournful and remained bereaved. When Kevin recovered, he still did not overcome his sorrow!

One day Kevin applied for a vacancy. The Applicant got the job to his complete surprise. A temporary position. A Library Assistant. The Temp worked for only six weeks. Finally, at the end of his temporary Employment, that Employment was terminated.

From the Employee being rejected by the Employer,

Kevin become suicidal. He attempted to commit suicide by taking a drug overdose. In an Ambulance, the patient was rushed to Hospital. He was pumped out. For Nights and Days, Kevin recuperated, recovered and convalesced. Kevin was a convalescent during his time of convalescence at home. With sanity, he fought for his deliverance. Kevin gained redemption and salvation. He became converted to a Christian!

Kevin ended up becoming a devout Christian. From his Christian Faith Kevin was devoted. The Christian had a devotion to Christ!

Kevin possessed a charismatic gift that the Christian was bestowed with. Actually, as things unveiled, the Christian also did have charisma!

# 1
# KEVIN'S DETENTION

Kevin was detained after school. He attended his detention. Sitting down at a table in the middle of the classroom, the pupil wrote out lines about a hundred times.

I MUSTN'T TALK IN CLASS.

That school day, Kevin came home later than usual. His Mother Patty showed concern for her punished son.

"What time do you call this? Where have you been?"

"Mom, I am sorry I am late. I had a detention," apologised son.

"What did you get in trouble for this time?" enquired Mother.

"Sir said no talking in class. Me, I talked in class."

"You must shut that gob of yours," scowled Mother.

"It wasn't my intention to talk. I just talked anyway," said Kevin calmly.

"Now that you're here. Go to your room and say your prayers," demanded Mother.

"Do I have to?" objected son.

Patty enforced discipline.

"Do as you are told. I'll give you a clip around the earhole."

Kevin, obeying his Mother, left the lounge. He went upstairs to his bedroom. He entered his bedroom alone. He knelt down by his bed there on a rug. He began to pray. He struggled to say a prayer.

"Please, Lord! I don't understand. Help me do right! I need you right now. I can't cope. Please help me! I need your love and your guidance," pleaded Kevin.

As a punishment, Patty did not cook for her son. Kevin skipped a meal. His supper. Kevin did not watch television. He stayed in his bedroom for hours and hours. For several hours, Kevin relaxed, recuperated, rested and meditated.

That night, Kevin went straight to bed at the usual time.

Tomorrow morning attending school.

# 2
# DAYDREAMER

During the Religious Education lesson, Kevin daydreamed by looking out of the window dreamily. The schoolboy engaged in daydreaming. A daydreamer.

The stern schoolteacher called out to a dreamy Kevin who sitting, stirred from his position. Moving position, Kevin looked at the experienced schoolteacher standing opposite him.

"Kevin, what's your denomination?" asked Mr Brady.

"Sir. My parents are both Catholics. I don't think I am," replied Kevin.

Sitting at tables nearby a few schoolgirls raised their arms in the air gracefully. The Irish ones proudly proclaimed themselves as Catholics unashamedly.

"We are Catholics. We believe," they said proudly.

The attentive schoolteacher showed favour to them. The schoolteacher had a certain favouritism for one of the pupils.

"Good!" praised Mr Brady.

In the classroom, all of the other pupils sitting at tables were mostly indifferent to Roman Catholicism. They may have had an indifference to the Religion.

The ones who were proud Catholics proclaimed with pride. They showed patriotism. The class did their classwork. The topic was Religion.

Kevin remained apathetic about this subject. This subject remained compulsory. The pupil tried to understand the subject. It's of a spiritual nature.

Leaving the classroom, Kevin made his way to the Science block. He walked past crowds of schoolchildren going through the corridors. Kevin attended science. He learned about various sciences. He disliked science because of being typically innumerate. Sitting at the very front of the Laboratory he appeared utterly bored with Physics. It's a complex subject. It's rather too complicated. Kevin could not grasp the subject matter. It was too difficult for him. Every pupil in this class was of average ability in Physics. (A member of his Form excelled in Physics. Surpassing everybody else.)

The schoolteacher gave back their tests to everybody in the class.

Every pupil looked at theirs. Kevin looked at his test result. He had failed his test. He obtained a low mark.

After the school bell had gone, the Physics lesson had ended. Kevin put his things quickly in his sports bag.

Hurriedly the pupil left the Science block. Going out of a main entrance. There in the school grounds, he lounged about at break time. At that time there were other cold pupils in groups shivering while talking.

Kevin, a pupil felt lonely, miserable and unhappy.

Standing near a school building there were different entrances. It was triangular. It looked like a triangle. It had an angular shape.

Kevin walked around the school grounds everywhere. He passed by the blocks, buildings and departments.

There, somewhere else in the school grounds, he saw a few schoolgirls in a group talking. Kevin ogled a schoolgirl. Kevin desired one of them. He fancied her. But that particular schoolgirl undesired and unloved him. He still remained ambivalent to most Females nowadays. Feeling unhappy, he lacked interest in attending his next period. Finally, in the end, Kevin decided to skive off school.

Later at home, Kevin was all alone. He watched a video nasty which he borrowed from a friend of his. Due to boredom, he watched it. Afterwards, Kevin hid the video as a protective measure. The prospect of it being banned remained a certain possibility.

That night Kevin had a bad nightmare!


Kevin's Brother, Graham Nally, came home at the weekend after staying the night at a friend's house. Kevin was pleased to see his Brother. Both Brothers stayed together in the lounge. They both conversed with each other.

"How was it at your friend's?" asked Kevin.

"It was alright. I watched videos," replied Brother.

"I watched a video too," mumbled Kevin.

"What was it about?" asked Brother.

"It's about a flesh-eating monster in space," answered Kevin.

"You shouldn't be watching that. Don't give up on your religion," cautioned Brother.

With scepticism and disbelief, he had doubted the Catholic Religion.

"What's the point? I don't believe. I don't have faith," said Kevin unashamedly.

"Our Mother is sort of Catholic. Why don't you follow her principles?" paused Brother. "And our Gran is full of wisdom."

An unbeliever and sceptic, Kevin deeply thought of his Grandmother, Franny Nally. Kevin respected Grandmother's wisdom. He had high regard for his Grandmother.

"I don't understand her old wives' tales. Nor do I get her Irish Folklore," murmured Kevin.

Graham regarded his Grandmother as a sweet blessing.

"Franny is a blessing," praised Graham. "So says Mother."

Kevin tried to fathom the mystery.

"Do you think Franny is a blessing in disguise?" perplexed Kevin.

"I believe so. Gran is full of wisdom."

"Maybe Granny can help. I am down. I failed my exams. I worry. What am I going to do? What prospects do I have?" frowned Kevin.

"Listen to Mom. Say your prayers," advised Brother.

Kevin got up. Leaving his Brother in a downstairs room.

Kevin went upstairs and stayed in his bedroom. There he isolated himself. He suffered from a bout of depression. Kevin stayed in his bedroom for many hours until he finally went to bed that night.

A few nights later, Kevin stayed up and watched a gothic horror on television. An Irish Folklore. The Little Red Riding Hood legend. Very late at night-time. Was Kevin possessed? Was he under possession?

# 3
# KEVIN'S FOOTBALL DISAPPOINTMENTS

One afternoon, the many schoolboys played football on the playing field on a football pitch, for their P.E. lesson. That day the weather was fine.

Three Forms played each other at football. Kevin and his Form played badly in their first game. The team lost the game.

On their second game, Kevin's team were thrashed by the eventual (winners) winning team.

The disappointed team trudge off the football pitch when going back to a pavilion.

Kevin's hopes for playing for the school football team were dashed. And everyone else's hopes and aspirations too.

Kevin lost his desire to play football then. He would probably give it up. Kevin was once noted for his good strong tackles as a defender.

Coming home, Kevin isolated himself. Kevin felt very disappointed. He still hadn't overcome his disappointment. Kevin stayed in his untidy bedroom and rested.

Later that night, Graham came into his younger

Brother's bedroom. Graham an older Brother intruded on his Brother.

"C'mon. Aren't you going to watch the match with me? It's on," prompted Brother.

Kevin made a gesture.

"No. You go and watch it. I think I'll stay here," said Kevin unenthusiastically.

Graham then left his deeply unhappy and miserable Brother.

Graham went downstairs to watch European football on television. Graham a fan had a passion for football.

Meanwhile, Kevin lost his enthusiasm for football, especially tonight. He still remained unenthusiastic about it. He gave it up and pursued an alternative interest.

# 4
# KEVIN SUFFERS WITH MISERY

For most periods the Female pupils shunned, ignored and rejected Kevin a schoolboy. They undesired and unloved him. They may have thought of him as being unappealing, undesirable and working class.

Kevin developed no relationship or friendship with regard to any of them. He despised and disliked them.

None of the Female pupils really bothered to talk to him either in his Form or in class.

During his school days, these pupils may have been average. All were destined to fail!

Kevin deemed himself a failure! He made no progress in his education. (His school report was rather bad.)

Usually, Kevin was a loner. A lonely schoolboy. Naturally, he was spurned by everybody.

Perhaps because he was Irish? A dunce at school!

Kevin Nally did desire an irresistible schoolgirl whom he fancied! But time after time he was naturally rejected by them.

As Kevin grew older in his adolescence things did change. A few Females showed interest and love towards him. Their delightful charmed smiles were so sweet. On different schooldays, there were different schoolgirls and a tall Sixth Former sat next to Kevin on a crowded Bus of passengers.

They all showed such deep love towards him. They had been so nice, sweet and amiable to Kevin.

# 5
# PATTY FORCES HER SON TO TIDY UP BEDROOM

Patty burst into her son's untidy bedroom. Patty forced her son to tidy up his bedroom.

"Son. Tidy up your bedroom now. It is a mess," demanded Mother.

Kevin disobeyed his Mother. He remained stubborn. A wayward and disobedient Teenager.

Patty in anger shouted at her son.

"Do as you are told. Tidy up your bedroom now. Do it!"

The son obeyed his Mother. Kevin tidied up his bedroom. He sorted out everything neatly. His piles of books, clothes, cassettes and videos on the dirty carpet.

Kevin changed his linen. He put clean bedsheets on his bed. He dusted his bedroom. He also polished the table and cleaned the window sills. He hoovered the carpet thoroughly. As soon as Kevin had finished cleaning up his bedroom, Patty came and inspected her son's bedroom. Patty approved of it. Now Kevin's nice bedroom was clean and tidy. Patty stopped nagging her son. Patty left her moody son to calm down.

Much later, Kevin spent time doing his homework.

Kevin did his homework.

Later in the evening, Kevin was all alone at home.

Kevin desired a human Female's love!

So, to overcome his burning desire and obsessive infatuation, he spent time watching a soft porn video. Kevin engaged in his sexual fantasies.

# 6
# KEVIN'S OBSESSIONAL FAVOURITES

Kevin took an interest in watching various videos of his choice. His favourite preference remained comedy films, science fiction films, sleuth films and thrillers.

He got corrupted and depraved at watching horror films and salacious movies. (He had a tendency for watching pornographic films. He tended to satisfy his fantasy desires which he engaged to stimulate with pornographic stimulus.)

At home, Kevin usually watched horror films and soft porn films whenever his Mother was not in.

Straightaway he hid the videos away.

Kevin a teenage schoolboy grew up to be deprived, depraved, corrupt and prurient. His prurience was that of a schoolboy, a Teenager developing from puberty.

From having an interest in watching videos and films, Kevin was fully aware that sooner or later he would be found out. How could he explain himself? His passion for films. Watching really bad movies such as horrors and pornography for instance.

Sinning, Kevin had felt unashamed of himself. With hardly any conscience.

# 7
# MUSIC LAST PERIOD

Kevin wandered through the school grounds with purposeful intent. He tried to look for any of them. He felt eager with desire. Suddenly, he saw desirable schoolgirls whom he desired. Standing in a group near the flowerbed.

One of them did not mix with commoners. They unnoticed the plebeian.

Kevin had a crush on Edwina with infatuation desired Edwina but Edwina snubbed and shunned commoners. Kevin wanted to talk to Edwina but he felt too nervous and shy in the presence of her schoolfellows. Kevin made no impression on any of them. He unimpressed them. They appeared to be condescending towards the vulnerable schoolboy. Kevin felt humiliated, hurt and unhappy again. Suffering with misery. He remained a loner. A lonely schoolboy sitting on a bench all alone at a far corner of a brick wall near the entrance to the Science Block.

Later as the school bell went, the pupils, Forms attended their Registration in their Form Room.

Apparently moody, miserable and unhappy Kevin remained silent during Form Registration. The Form was punctual for their attendance of Registration.

For the very last two periods, Kevin attended his lessons.

For the last period, the Music class enjoyed singing as their Music Teacher sat and played the piano. It was a good singsong. Most definitely an enjoyable experience. An emotive one!

(Kevin felt apathetic about music lessons. But he did love listening to music.)

Kevin experienced a last lesson in Music to be highly enjoyable, exciting and too soulful!

This pupil never felt as happy as this before. It remained a strange experience. A wonderful one too!

This last period rounded off the shortened school day. (There earlier today was a School Assembly held in a Hall. Attended by all Forms.)

# 8
# LONELINESS

At the weekend on a nice sunny day, Kevin mowed the lawn out in the back garden. He mowed it in beautiful straight, horizontal lines. Afterwards, he put away the lawnmower in the garage.

Going to the back door doorstep at the back of the semi-detached house, he took off his trainers. He put on his plimsols. Kevin entered indoors.

Kevin joined his Brother in the lounge. His studious Brother, an Apprentice was too engrossed in reading a Manual.

Kevin sat down in an armchair at the far corner of the room. Next to a sideboard. There he rested.

Sitting in a corner of the settee, Graham had been distracted by his younger Brother entering. Graham glanced up.

"You should be a Gardener. You have done a good job on the garden," remarked Brother.

"I like gardening. I don't know about that," said Kevin miserably.

Graham observed his sullen Brother in a mood.

"Why are you gloomy?" asked Brother.

"No one seems to love me. How about you?"

"I have a girlfriend. It is steady," answered Brother.

Kevin envied his elder Brother. Graham's fortune was a blessing!

"You're lucky," said Kevin enviously.

Kevin feeling envious got up and left the lounge. Suffering from depression and loneliness.

He stayed in his bedroom for hours until he had recuperated. He fully rested during that time.

Kevin dreaded going to school on a Monday!

# 9
# LOSING HER COOL, GRANDMOTHER REPRIMANDED KEVIN

The elderly Grandmother entered the lounge. Grandmother steadily walked while holding a walking stick. Unthinkingly, Grandmother stooped down to eject a video cassette from the cassette recorder.

"Don't watch this! It's bad! Stop it at once," reprimanded Grandmother.

Kevin was annoyed at his Grandmother for spoiling his enjoyment of watching a bawdy film.

"I want to watch the film," grumbled Kevin.

"How many times have I told you? Don't watch this! Do watch good films. Not bad films," cautioned Grandmother.

Kevin was disobedient and stubborn.

"Can't I watch it?" moaned Kevin.

Grandmother agitated Kevin for his lack of morality.

"Where are your morals? Why aren't you a Catholic like me?" questioned Grandmother.

"You are a Catholic. You have wisdom," acknowledged Kevin.

"I don't want to see you watching any bad videos.

Do you hear me? Have I made myself clear?" reprimanded Grandmother.

Kevin remained set in his teenage ways and disobeyed his Grandmother.

He remained disobedient. (With immediate effect Kevin did listen to his Grandmother trying to caution and discipline him.)

Grandmother held a rosary in her hand.

"Kevin. My dear! Don't watch bad videos or bad television. Look at good things. Be a Catholic. Follow the Catholic way. I do. Your Mother tries. So why don't you?"

Although Kevin did listen to his Grandmother, he still watched bad videos and bad films on television as usual.

# 10
# KEVIN'S DESIRE

Kevin went to a sweet shop in a street. There he saw on display racks of blue movies, and soft porn videos. Kevin wanted to take out a pornographic video. He was very tempted. Actually, having a temptation urge to do it. The video cover was erotic. The tanned nude Blonde aroused him. He became excited with desire.

Kevin was a Teenager growing up and going through an adolescent phase of watching pornography. He became rather interested in watching porn videos, films and blue movies collectively.

Kevin hurriedly left the corner sweet shop. He walked home to his house within reach. At his house, he found himself all alone at home. The only one who remained indoors. Kevin got bored of doing nothing. He decided to watch a video to occupy his time. (Watching films remained an enjoyable interest of his.)

So, he inserted a blue movie in the video recorder which he had previously borrowed from a friend of his. He watched pornography. Kevin satisfied his carnal desires and sexual fantasies. The schoolboy's ones!

Kevin felt quite unfulfilled again. Kevin craved more. He longed for the one he loved!

Going to bed late, that night Kevin had a wet dream!

# 11
# KEVIN'S NERVOUS BREAKDOWNS TO HIS FINAL CONVERSION

During May at secondary school, Kevin a candidate sat his C.S.E. Examinations and in the Summer Term, he sat his G.C.E. Examinations in an Examination Hall. (Kevin had been entered for private entrance for two G.C.E. subjects.)

In the next school year, during the Autumn Term, the humiliated, frustrated and embarrassed Sixth Former enrolled for the Sixth Form.

The following summer (TERM) Kevin failed his G.C.E. EXAMINATIONS.

At home, an unsympathetic Patty nagged her son for failing his Examinations.

In the Autumn, Kevin enrolled in college. Kevin failed his Examinations again.

As a result, Kevin had no prospects for Education and Employment. He still remained unemployed in modern society.

In his miserable and depressed state of mind, Kevin still continued to watch porn and horror films alone by himself. His miseries afflicted him!

## Kevin

One day, Kevin somehow got a job interview. Kevin attended a job interview at Personnel. To his complete surprise, he got the job to work at a toy Department in a Department store. The Employee's start date for this Retail Assistant position was Monday morning. (Applying for the vacancy and getting the job buoyed Kevin up.) A temporary position.

On Saturday afternoon, a lovely witch came over to see his Mother.

Subsequently, Erica invited Kevin to her house. There Kevin met Erica's Husband and their two blonde sons. Later, he met a playful Teenage Girl. The Daughter Erica's Friend was a gorgeous Brunette.

Suddenly Kevin was becoming insane. Was he possessed by evil spirits? He was frightened of witchcraft and from being in the presence of a witch's coven. Kevin's ignorance of the black arts, black magic and witchcraft made him a victim!

Kevin was driven mad by fear. He was frightened. In a fearful state.

Erica and her close friend, a passenger, came along with her. Erica drove Kevin a passenger home. Kevin ended up having a nervous breakdown. He was insane.

Kevin was taken to his G.P. Then he was admitted to Hospital in a Psychiatric Unit. Kevin was feeling suicidal because he did not start his new job!

From his admittance to Hospital the patient was sectioned.

Going insane the Psychiatric Patient escaped a ward and ran away in his hospital pyjamas. The carers caught the deranged patient. The patient was taken back to a locked-up ward under supervision. The patient was injected, sedated and drugged up. On certain days he had more blood tests administered over the course of the weeks.

The patient sat down in the company of other patients in a ward. Kevin felt anxious, fearful, frightened and too sad. He tried to read his pocket Bible. He may have been a zealot.

At that time, the professional Nurses on duty attended to Kevin. The Nurses wearing uniforms nursed him back to health. Another one showed deep concern for the patient.

At night, the patient took his medication which was forced on him. Every Wednesday morning Kevin attended Occupational Therapy. (On one morning Kevin did cooking with a small group. He ate a meal with everyone else at the kitchen table in the modern kitchen.)

During visiting hours, the visitors who visited Kevin at hospital at the ward were usually his Mother, Sister and Pastor.

During Kevin's long stay at Hospital in a ward, the patient saw professionals. This patient was seen at a ward round. The Consulting Team of Health

Professionals attending the consultation were all present.

Finally, after his section elapsed, the patient was discharged from Hospital. Kevin recovered. In the future probably a relapse was inevitable.

Months later, Kevin began to write stories. Kevin felt vulnerable as well as exposed to witchcraft. He developed a talent for writing.

About a year ago, Kevin's best friend died. Kevin was heartbroken, mournful and bereaved. He grieved for his friend.

Going to church one night, a churchgoer rescued Kevin. At church the very small group which came. Together they played a child's game. This could have been a turning point to Kevin's future conversion!

Then one day an Applicant applied for a vacancy. Somehow Kevin got the job. This job was a temporary position as an Assistant Librarian at a central Library.

After about six weeks of temporary employment, Kevin was rejected by the Manager. Unfortunately, his Application had been rejected. It had not been taken up any further by Personnel. The Applicant's rejection of the Application had been disappointing!

From rejection and becoming suicidal, Kevin

attempted to commit suicide by trying to drown himself in a filled-up bath of hot bath water and at another time with a drug overdose!

At a hospital in a bed, the patient had a tube forced down in his mouth. The patient had been pumped out. All of the drugs. The suffering patient had felt a deep firm pressure applied to his Trachea which gave a vibrating painful effect. The acute pain was excruciating. The hospitalised patient suffering from pain. Kevin convalesced.

Living at home with his Mother, he spent time convalescing.

Long ago, Kevin had another relapse again and a breakdown.

Kevin was admitted to Hospital again. From the patient's admittance this time Kevin was sectioned again.

After less than a month of his stay in hospital, in a Psychiatric Unit, Ward, the patient was discharged from Hospital. Now he was a discharged patient referred to outpatients.

Subsequently, Kevin become converted. The sinner and repenter gained salvation.

Eventually, Kevin become a devout Christian. He was devoted. He had a devotion to the Lord. The Christian sought redemption.

Kevin, unemployed ultimately possessed a charismatic gift. He was bestowed with a gift. He possessed such great charisma!

Kevin finally found peace and joy at last in his peaceful life!

Kevin took great comfort in having freedom. From his condition, Kevin was free from possession. He realised from spiritual experience that life itself is spiritual warfare. Ultimately, he became familiar with reading Revelations. Kevin gained revelational enlightenment and illumination by studying Revelations. At home in a study.

Kevin fully understood the true significance of spiritual warfare. The ignorant Christian learning tried to fathom the mysteries.

Kevin did gain spiritual knowledge and wisdom by learning the scriptures and teaching. His Christian Faith protected him from evil.

The Christian's good faith developed with spirituality, knowledge, wisdom and experience. He acquired gifts, spiritual ones too. (Spiritual Discernment etc.)

Life for Kevin was much happier, peaceful and joyful as a Christian, and a believer.

The Christian became formidable and invincible in his Faith in the Lord. The Christian's Faith grew strong in the Lord. A devotion. His love for Christ was a beatitude!

Kevin developed a deep spirituality. He had a spiritual sense. Kevin possessed an intuition. An intuitive intellect. Spiritually, his battle was a spiritual warfare.

Kevin was an aesthete, connoisseur and artist. (He had a passion for writing. The process of creative writing was something he enjoyed doing.)

Kevin undertook a project of his but he failed to get his work published. His ambition was to become a professional writer. Kevin remained ambitious. (He did fail in his aspirations for everything else.)

Once the student dropped out of college at least twice in two TOURISM COURSES. The student felt humiliated at finding a gorgeous uniformed Employee of a Travel Agent at college.

Eventually, Kevin got educated. Ultimately, Kevin pursued a career as a Professional Writer. Getting published was a motivational objective. Whether he succeeded or not remained immaterial. The Author dreamt of being a great writer. The Author was immortal. The Author's conquest for immortality was only a dream!

- THE END -

*Available worldwide from Amazon
and all good bookstores*

---

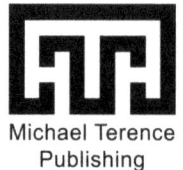

www.mtp.agency

www.facebook.com/mtp.agency

@mtp_agency

www.ingramcontent.com/pod-product-compliance
Lightning Source LLC
LaVergne TN
LVHW051218070526
838200LV00063B/4949